Managing Type 2 Diabetes: Practical Strategies for a Healthier Lifestyle.

Empowering Yourself Through Diet, Exercise, and Lifestyle Changes

Dr. Maggie Alkaline

ISBN: 9798325719752

Acknowledgement

I extend my heartfelt gratitude to all those who have contributed to the creation of this book, "Managing Type 2 Diabetes: Practical Strategies for a Healthier Lifestyle."
To my family, whose unwavering support and encouragement have been my source of strength throughout this journey. Your patience and understanding during the long hours spent researching and writing are deeply appreciated.
To my colleagues and mentors in the field of endocrinology, thank you for sharing your knowledge and expertise, which have enriched the content of this book.
To the healthcare professionals and individuals living with diabetes who have generously shared their experiences and insights, your stories have added depth and authenticity to the narrative.
To the publishing team, editors, and designers who have worked tirelessly to bring this book to life, thank you for your dedication and professionalism.

CONTENTS

EPIGRAPH

"In the midst of chaos, there is also opportunity."

Sun Tzu

DEDICATION

To all those who have bravely faced the challenges of managing type 2 diabetes, may this book serve as a beacon of hope and empowerment on your journey to a healthier and happier life. Your resilience and determination inspire us all.

Introduction

Welcome to "Managing Type 2 Diabetes: Practical Strategies for a Healthier Lifestyle." In this introductory chapter, we delve into the fundamentals of understanding Type 2 diabetes, a prevalent chronic condition affecting millions worldwide.

1. Understanding Type 2 Diabetes

Type 2 diabetes is a metabolic disorder characterized by high blood sugar levels due to either insufficient insulin production or the body's inability to effectively utilize insulin. Unlike Type 1 diabetes, which typically manifests in childhood and is caused by the immune system attacking insulin-producing cells, Type 2 diabetes often develops later in life and is closely connected to existence factors such as diet, physical activity, and obesity.

One of the defining features of Type 2 diabetes is insulin resistance, wherein the body's cells become less responsive to insulin's effects, leading to elevated blood sugar levels. Over time, this can result in various complications affecting the heart, kidneys, eyes, nerves, and other organs.

I. The Prevalence and Impact of Type 2 Diabetes

The prevalence of Type 2 diabetes has reached epidemic proportions globally, with an estimated 463 million adults aged 20-79 living with the condition in 2019. This number is projected to rise to 700 million by 2045 if current trends persist. The burden of Type 2 diabetes extends beyond individual health, placing significant strain on healthcare systems and economies worldwide.

Type 2 diabetes is associated with an increased risk of cardiovascular disease, stroke, kidney disease, blindness, lower limb amputations, and premature death. The economic costs associated with treating diabetes and its complications are staggering, accounting for billions in healthcare expenditures annually.

II. Risk Factors for Type 2 Diabetes

While genetics play a role in predisposing individuals to Type 2 diabetes, lifestyle factors exert significant influence over disease development and progression.

Key risk factors include:

1.   Obesity: Excess body weight, particularly abdominal adiposity, increases the risk of insulin resistance and Type 2 diabetes.

2.   Physical Inactivity: Sedentary lifestyles contribute to insulin resistance and impair glucose metabolism, raising the risk of Type 2 diabetes.

3.   Unhealthy Diet: Diets high in refined carbohydrates, sugars, saturated fats, and processed foods can contribute to obesity, insulin resistance, and elevated blood sugar levels.

4.   Family History: Having a close family member with Type 2 diabetes increases one's risk of developing the condition.

5.   Age: The risk of Type 2 diabetes increases with age, particularly after 45 years old.

III.   The Role of Lifestyle in Type 2 Diabetes Management

While genetic predisposition plays a role in Type 2 diabetes risk, lifestyle factors such as diet, physical activity, stress management, and sleep patterns exert significant influence over disease development and progression. Adopting healthy lifestyle habits can mitigate risk factors, improve glycemic control, and reduce the likelihood of diabetes-related complications.

Conclusion

In this introductory chapter, we've explored the fundamentals of Type 2 diabetes, including its definition, prevalence, impact, risk factors, and the critical role of lifestyle in disease management. Understanding the complexities of Type 2 diabetes is the first step toward effective prevention and management. Throughout this ebook, we'll delve deeper into practical strategies and evidence-based recommendations to empower individuals with Type 2 diabetes to take control of their health and well-being.

Join us on this journey as we navigate the challenges of managing Type 2 diabetes and explore strategies for achieving a healthier lifestyle.

2. Importance of Lifestyle Changes

Type 2 diabetes is a complex metabolic disorder influenced by a myriad of factors, including genetics, environment, and lifestyle choices. While genetics may predispose individuals to diabetes, lifestyle factors play a significant role in its development and progression. Adopting healthy lifestyle changes is paramount in managing Type 2 diabetes and reducing the risk of complications.

I.   Dietary Modifications

One of the most impactful lifestyle changes for individuals with Type 2 diabetes is dietary modification. A balanced diet that focuses on whole, unprocessed foods such as fruits, vegetables, lean proteins, whole grains, and healthy fats can help regulate blood sugar levels, improve insulin sensitivity, and promote overall health. Monitoring carbohydrate intake, especially refined sugars and simple carbohydrates, is essential for managing blood glucose levels.

II.   Regular Physical Activity

Physical activity is another cornerstone of diabetes management. Exercise helps lower blood sugar levels by increasing insulin sensitivity and promoting the uptake of glucose by muscles for energy. Regular aerobic exercise, such as brisk walking, cycling, swimming, or dancing, can improve cardiovascular health, aid in weight management, and reduce the risk of complications associated with Type 2 diabetes.

III.   Weight Management

Maintaining a healthy weight is crucial for managing Type 2 diabetes, as excess body fat, particularly around the abdomen, can worsen insulin resistance and increase the risk of complications. Adopting a calorie-controlled diet, engaging in regular physical activity, and incorporating strength training exercises to build lean muscle mass can help individuals achieve and maintain a healthy weight.

IV.   Stress Reduction and Sleep Hygiene

Chronic stress and poor sleep quality can negatively impact blood sugar control and exacerbate diabetes-related complications. Practicing stress-reduction techniques such as mindfulness meditation, deep breathing exercises, and yoga can help manage stress levels and promote emotional well-being. Additionally, prioritizing good sleep hygiene by maintaining a regular sleep schedule, creating a relaxing bedtime routine, and optimizing sleep environment can improve sleep quality and support overall health.

Conclusion

In conclusion, lifestyle changes play a pivotal role in managing Type 2 diabetes and improving overall health outcomes. By adopting a healthy diet, engaging in regular physical activity, managing stress, and prioritizing sleep, individuals with Type 2 diabetes can take proactive steps towards better management of their condition and reduce the risk of complications. Throughout this ebook, we will explore practical strategies and evidence-based recommendations to empower individuals with Type 2 diabetes to make sustainable lifestyle changes and achieve optimal health and well-being.

Chapter 2

Understanding Type 2 Diabetes (2)

In this chapter, we delve into the intricate mechanisms behind Type 2 diabetes, exploring its causes, risk factors, and underlying physiological processes.

1.   Causes and Risk Factors

Type 2 diabetes develops when the body becomes resistant to the effects of insulin or fails to produce enough insulin to maintain normal blood sugar levels. While the exact cause of Type 2 diabetes is multifactorial and not fully understood, several factors contribute to its development:

I.   **Genetic Predisposition**: Genetics plays a significant role in Type 2 diabetes risk, with certain genetic variations increasing susceptibility to the condition. Individuals with a family history of diabetes are at higher risk of developing the disease.

II.   **Obesity and Sedentary Lifestyle**: Excess body weight, particularly abdominal obesity, and physical inactivity are major contributors to insulin resistance and Type 2 diabetes. Adipose tissue, especially visceral fat, releases inflammatory cytokines and adipokines that disrupt insulin signaling and glucose metabolism.

III.   **Poor Diet**: Diets high in refined sugars, unhealthy fats, and processed foods contribute to insulin resistance and elevated blood sugar levels. Excessive consumption of sugary beverages, fast food, and processed snacks can lead to weight gain and metabolic dysfunction.

IV.   **Age and Ethnicity**: Advancing age is a significant risk factor for Type 2 diabetes, with the prevalence increasing substantially after age 45. Additionally, certain ethnic groups, including African Americans, Hispanic/Latino Americans, Native Americans, and Asian Americans, have a higher predisposition to the condition.

V.   **Gestational Diabetes**: Women who develop gestational diabetes during pregnancy are at increased risk of developing Type 2 diabetes later in life. Gestational diabetes indicates underlying insulin resistance and impaired glucose tolerance, which may persist beyond pregnancy.

VI. **Other Medical Conditions**: Certain medical conditions, such as polycystic ovary syndrome (PCOS), prediabetes, metabolic syndrome, and cardiovascular disease, are associated with an elevated risk of Type 2 diabetes.

Conclusion

Understanding the causes and risk factors of Type 2 diabetes is essential for early detection, prevention, and management of the condition. By addressing modifiable risk factors such as obesity, sedentary lifestyle, and poor diet, individuals can reduce their risk of developing Type 2 diabetes and improve overall health outcomes. In the subsequent sections of this ebook, we will explore strategies for

preventing and managing Type 2 diabetes through lifestyle modifications, dietary interventions, physical activity, and medication therapy.

2. Symptoms and Diagnosis

Type 2 diabetes often develops gradually, with subtle symptoms that may go unnoticed or be mistaken for other health issues. However, as the disease progresses, individuals may experience a constellation of symptoms indicative of abnormal glucose metabolism and insulin resistance. Common symptoms of Type 2 diabetes include:

I. Increased thirst and urination

Increased thirst and urination, medically known as polydipsia and polyuria, are common symptoms associated with Type 2 diabetes. These symptoms arise due to the body's inability to properly regulate blood sugar levels, leading to excessive urination and dehydration.

When blood sugar levels are high, the kidneys attempt to remove the excess glucose from the bloodstream by filtering it out into the urine. This process, known as glycosuria, results in increased urine production. As a consequence, individuals with Type 2 diabetes experience frequent urination, which can disrupt normal daily activities and sleep patterns.

Excessive urination can lead to dehydration, triggering the sensation of thirst as the body attempts to replenish lost fluids. Polydipsia, or increased thirst, is the body's natural response to fluid loss and dehydration. Individuals may find themselves drinking more fluids than usual in an attempt to quench their thirst and compensate for fluid losses.

Polydipsia and polyuria often occur together and can be early warning signs of undiagnosed diabetes. However, it's essential to note that these symptoms can also be indicative of other medical conditions, such as kidney disease or urinary tract infections. Therefore, anyone experiencing persistent thirst and frequent urination should seek medical evaluation to determine the underlying cause.

Managing polydipsia and polyuria in individuals with Type 2 diabetes typically involves controlling blood sugar levels through lifestyle modifications, including dietary changes, regular exercise, and medication therapy. By maintaining healthy blood sugar levels, individuals can alleviate symptoms of excessive thirst and urination and reduce the risk of complications associated with uncontrolled diabetes.

II.   Fatigue and weakness

Fatigue and weakness are common symptoms experienced by individuals with Type 2 diabetes and can significantly impact daily functioning and quality of life. These symptoms result from the body's inability to effectively utilize glucose for energy due to insulin resistance or insufficient insulin production.

In individuals with Type 2 diabetes, cells become resistant to the effects of insulin, a hormone responsible for facilitating the uptake of glucose from the bloodstream into cells to be used as fuel. As a result, glucose remains in the bloodstream, leading to elevated blood sugar levels. Without an adequate supply of glucose entering the cells, the body's tissues and organs, including muscles and brain, are deprived of energy, resulting in fatigue and weakness.

Additionally, fluctuations in blood sugar levels can contribute to feelings of fatigue and weakness. When blood sugar levels are too high, excess glucose is excreted in the urine, leading to dehydration and electrolyte imbalances, which can cause fatigue. Conversely, when blood sugar levels drop too low, a condition known as hypoglycemia, the brain and muscles may not receive enough glucose to function optimally, resulting in weakness and fatigue.

Furthermore, individuals with Type 2 diabetes often experience comorbidities such as obesity, high blood pressure, and cardiovascular disease, which can exacerbate feelings of fatigue and weakness. These conditions can place additional strain on the body and contribute to decreased energy levels.

Managing fatigue and weakness in individuals with Type 2 diabetes involves addressing the underlying factors contributing to these symptoms. This may include:

- **Blood sugar management**: Monitoring blood sugar levels regularly and following a balanced meal plan to help stabilize glucose levels.

Regular physical activity: Engaging in regular exercise can improve insulin sensitivity, enhance energy levels, and promote overall well-being.

- **Medication management**: Taking prescribed diabetes medications as directed by a healthcare provider to help regulate blood sugar levels.
- **Adequate sleep**: Ensuring sufficient rest and practicing good sleep hygiene can help combat fatigue and promote overall health.
- **Stress management**: Implementing stress-reduction techniques such as relaxation exercises, mindfulness, or counseling can help alleviate fatigue associated with emotional stress.
- **Nutritional support**: Consuming a nutrient-dense diet rich in fruits, vegetables, whole grains, lean proteins, and healthy fats can provide essential nutrients to support energy production and combat fatigue.

It's essential for individuals experiencing persistent fatigue and weakness to discuss these symptoms with a healthcare provider to determine the underlying cause and develop an appropriate treatment plan tailored to their needs. Addressing fatigue and weakness effectively can improve overall health and quality of life for individuals living with Type 2 diabetes.

- **Unintentional Weight Loss**: Despite increased appetite and calorie intake, some individuals with Type 2 diabetes may experience unintentional weight loss due to cellular starvation and breakdown of muscle and fat tissue. Weight loss may occur in conjunction with increased urinary excretion of calories, contributing to metabolic imbalance.
- **Blurred Vision**: High blood sugar levels can cause changes in the shape and flexibility of the lens in the eye, leading to blurred vision and difficulty focusing. Blurred vision is often temporary and resolves with adequate glucose control but may recur if blood sugar levels remain elevated.

- **Slow Wound Healing**: Diabetes-related vascular and immune dysfunction impair the body's ability to heal wounds and fight off infections. Minor cuts, bruises, and skin injuries may take longer to heal in individuals with Type 2 diabetes, increasing the risk of infection and complications.

III.   Diagnosis

The diagnosis of Type 2 diabetes is typically established through a combination of clinical evaluation, laboratory tests, and screening procedures. Diagnostic criteria for Type 2 diabetes include:

IV.   The Fasting Plasma Glucose

The Fasting Plasma Glucose (FPG) test is a blood test used to measure the concentration of glucose in the bloodstream after an overnight fast. It is one of the primary diagnostic tools for identifying diabetes and assessing glycemic control in individuals at risk of or living with the condition.

During the FPG test, the individual refrains from eating or drinking (except water) for at least 8 hours prior to the test. This fasting period ensures that any glucose present in the bloodstream is a result of endogenous production rather than recent dietary intake.

The test is typically performed in the morning after an overnight fast. A healthcare professional collects a blood sample from a vein in the arm using a needle and syringe or a fingerstick. The blood sample is then analyzed in a laboratory to determine the concentration of glucose.

V.   Interpretation of FPG results:

Normal: Fasting plasma glucose levels below 100 milligrams per deciliter (mg/dL) are considered normal.

Prediabetes: Fasting plasma glucose levels between 100 and 125 mg/dL indicate prediabetes, a condition characterized by impaired glucose tolerance and an increased risk of developing Type 2 diabetes.

Diabetes: Fasting plasma glucose levels of 126 mg/dL or higher on two separate occasions indicate diabetes.

The FPG test is valuable for diagnosing diabetes because it provides a snapshot of blood sugar levels in a fasted state, which reflects the body's ability to regulate glucose during periods of fasting. Elevated fasting plasma glucose levels indicate impaired fasting glucose metabolism, which may result from insulin resistance, impaired insulin secretion, or a combination of both.

In addition to diagnosing diabetes, the FPG test is used to monitor glycemic control in individuals with diabetes and assess the effectiveness of treatment interventions, including lifestyle modifications and medication therapy. Regular monitoring of fasting plasma glucose levels helps healthcare providers adjust treatment plans and optimize outcomes for individuals living with diabetes.

Overall, the FPG test is a critical tool in the diagnosis and management of diabetes, providing valuable insights into an individual's glucose metabolism and facilitating personalized care and treatment strategies.

Oral Glucose Tolerance Test (OGTT): In this test, individuals consume a glucose-rich beverage, and blood sugar levels are measured at regular intervals over several hours. A blood glucose level of 200 mg/dL or higher two hours after drinking the glucose solution confirms the diagnosis of diabetes.

Hemoglobin A1c (HbA1c) Test: The HbA1c test reflects average blood sugar levels over the past two to three months by measuring the percentage of glycated hemoglobin in the blood. An HbA1c level of 6.5% or higher is indicative of diabetes.

Conclusion

Recognizing the symptoms and diagnostic criteria for Type 2 diabetes is essential for timely intervention and management of the condition. Early detection allows for the implementation of lifestyle modifications, dietary changes, and medical therapy to improve glycemic control and prevent complications. In the subsequent sections of this ebook, we will delve into treatment options, self-management strategies, and preventive measures for individuals living with Type 2 diabetes.

3. Complications and Long-Term Effects

Type 2 diabetes is a chronic condition characterized by high blood sugar levels resulting from insulin resistance and inadequate insulin production. While managing blood sugar levels is crucial for preventing short-term complications such as hyperglycemia and hypoglycemia, it is equally important to understand the potential complications and long-term effects associated with Type 2 diabetes.

I.   Cardiovascular Complications:

Individuals with Type 2 diabetes are at increased risk of developing cardiovascular diseases such as coronary artery disease, heart attack, and stroke. High blood sugar levels can damage blood vessels and lead to atherosclerosis, a condition characterized by the buildup of plaque in the arteries, narrowing their diameter and reducing blood flow to vital organs. Over time, this can increase the risk of heart disease and stroke. Additionally, individuals with Type 2 diabetes often have comorbidities such as high blood pressure and dyslipidemia, further elevating their cardiovascular risk.

II.   Neuropathy:

Diabetic neuropathy is a common complication of Type 2 diabetes that affects the nerves, particularly those in the feet and legs. Over time, high blood sugar levels can damage the nerves, leading to symptoms such as numbness, tingling, burning pain, and weakness in the affected areas. Neuropathy can also impair sensation, making individuals with diabetes more prone to foot injuries and infections. Left untreated, diabetic neuropathy can progress to more severe complications such as foot ulcers, infections, and even amputation.

III.   Retinopathy:

Type 2 diabetes can also affect the eyes, leading to a condition known as diabetic retinopathy. High blood sugar levels can damage the blood vessels in the retina, the light-sensitive tissue at the back of the eye, causing them to leak fluid or bleed. This can result in vision problems such as blurred vision, floaters, and, in severe cases, vision loss. Regular eye exams are essential for detecting diabetic retinopathy early and preventing vision loss.

IV.   Nephropathy:

Diabetic nephropathy, or diabetic kidney disease, is a serious complication of Type 2 diabetes that affects the kidneys. High blood sugar levels can damage the small blood vessels in the kidneys, impairing their ability to filter waste products from the blood effectively. Over time, this can lead to kidney damage and ultimately kidney failure, requiring dialysis or kidney transplantation. Individuals with Type 2 diabetes should undergo regular screening tests to assess kidney function and detect nephropathy early.

V.   Peripheral Arterial Disease (PAD):

Peripheral arterial disease is a condition characterized by narrowed arteries in the legs and feet, reducing blood flow to these areas. Individuals with Type 2 diabetes are at increased risk of developing PAD due to the damaging effects of high blood sugar levels on blood vessels. Symptoms of PAD include leg pain, cramping, numbness, and weakness, particularly during physical activity. PAD can also increase the risk of foot ulcers and amputation in individuals with diabetes.

VI.   Mental Health Effects:

Living with Type 2 diabetes can also impact mental health, leading to increased rates of depression, anxiety, and diabetes-related distress. The challenges of managing a chronic condition, coping with potential complications, and adhering to complex treatment regimens can take a toll on emotional well-being. It is essential for individuals with Type 2 diabetes to prioritize self-care, seek support from healthcare providers and mental health professionals, and engage in activities that promote overall well-being.

VII.   Quality of Life:

The complications and long-term effects of Type 2 diabetes can significantly impact an individual's quality of life, affecting their physical health, emotional well-being, and daily functioning. Managing diabetes effectively through lifestyle modifications, medication management, and regular medical care can help minimize the risk of complications and improve overall quality of life. However, it is essential for individuals with Type 2 diabetes to remain vigilant about monitoring their health, adhering to treatment recommendations, and seeking prompt medical attention for any concerning symptoms or changes in health status.

In summary, understanding the potential complications and long-term effects associated with Type 2 diabetes is crucial for individuals living with this condition. By actively managing blood sugar levels, adopting a healthy lifestyle, and seeking regular medical care, individuals with Type 2 diabetes can reduce their risk of complications and improve their overall health and well-being.

Chapter 3

Taking Control of Your Health. focus on the below.

1. Building a Support System

Building a support system is essential for individuals with Type 2 diabetes to effectively manage their health and well-being. A support system provides encouragement, guidance, and practical assistance in navigating the challenges associated with diabetes management. Whether it's family members, friends, healthcare professionals, or community resources, having a strong support network can make a significant difference in one's ability to take control of their health.

I.   Family Support:

Family members play a crucial role in supporting individuals with Type 2 diabetes. They can offer emotional support, help with meal planning and preparation, encourage physical activity, and provide assistance with medication management. In addition, family members can participate in educational programs and healthcare appointments to better understand diabetes and how to support their loved ones effectively. Open communication and collaboration within the family are key to creating a supportive environment conducive to diabetes management.

II.   Friends and Peers:

Friends and peers can also provide valuable support to individuals with Type 2 diabetes. They can offer encouragement, share experiences, and provide practical tips for managing diabetes in various social and lifestyle settings. Joining support groups or online communities for individuals with diabetes can help individuals connect with others who understand their challenges and can offer empathy, advice, and encouragement. Peer support can help reduce feelings of isolation and provide a sense of belonging and camaraderie.

III.   Healthcare Team:

Healthcare professionals play a critical role in supporting individuals with

Type 2 diabetes in managing their health. This may include primary care physicians, endocrinologists, diabetes educators, dietitians, nurses, pharmacists, and other specialists. These healthcare providers can offer medical expertise, personalized treatment recommendations, and ongoing monitoring of diabetes-related health parameters. Regular healthcare appointments allow individuals to discuss their concerns, track their progress, and receive guidance on optimizing their diabetes management plan.

IV.   Diabetes Education Programs:

Diabetes education programs provide individuals with Type 2 diabetes with the knowledge and skills necessary to manage their condition effectively. These programs cover topics such as nutrition, physical activity, medication management, blood sugar monitoring, and complication prevention. Participants learn practical strategies for making healthy lifestyle choices, coping with diabetes-related challenges, and navigating healthcare systems. Diabetes education programs may be offered through healthcare facilities, community organizations, or online platforms.

V.   Community Resources:

Community resources can complement formal healthcare services by providing additional support and resources for individuals with Type 2 diabetes. This may include local wellness programs, exercise classes, cooking demonstrations, support groups, and health fairs. Community organizations such as churches, schools, and nonprofit organizations may offer diabetes prevention and management initiatives tailored to the needs of their communities. Accessing community resources can help individuals with Type 2 diabetes find additional support and opportunities for healthy living.

VI.   Online Resources:

The internet offers a wealth of information and resources for individuals with Type 2 diabetes seeking support and guidance. Online platforms provide access to educational materials, interactive tools, peer support forums, and virtual coaching programs. Individuals can access reliable information on diabetes management, connect with others facing similar challenges, and access self-management tools to track their progress. However, it's essential to ensure that online resources are credible and evidence-based to avoid misinformation.

VII.   Self-Care Practices:

In addition to external support systems, individuals with Type 2 diabetes can also engage in self-care practices to support their health and well-being. This may include prioritizing adequate sleep, managing stress through relaxation techniques or mindfulness practices, engaging in regular physical activity, and practicing healthy eating habits. Self-care allows individuals to take an active role in managing their diabetes and promoting overall health and well-being.

In conclusion,

building a support system is essential for individuals with Type 2 diabetes to effectively manage their health and well-being. By cultivating supportive relationships with family, friends, healthcare professionals, and community resources, individuals can access the guidance, encouragement, and practical assistance they need to navigate the challenges of diabetes management successfully. A strong support system can empower individuals with Type 2 diabetes to take control of their health and live well with their condition.

2. Setting Realistic Goals

Setting realistic goals is a fundamental aspect of taking control of one's health, especially for individuals with Type 2 diabetes. By establishing achievable objectives, individuals can effectively manage their condition, improve their overall health, and enhance their quality of life. Setting realistic goals involves careful consideration of personal capabilities, priorities, and resources, as well as collaboration with healthcare professionals to develop a tailored action plan. In this chapter, we explore the importance of setting realistic goals in managing Type 2 diabetes and provide practical strategies for goal setting and implementation.

I.   Understanding the Importance of Goal Setting:

Setting goals provides individuals with Type 2 diabetes with a clear direction and purpose for their health-related efforts. Goals serve as benchmarks for progress, motivation for behavior change, and indicators of success. By defining specific, measurable, achievable, relevant, and time-bound (SMART) goals, individuals can create a roadmap for managing their diabetes effectively and making sustainable lifestyle changes. Goal setting also fosters accountability and empowerment, as individuals take ownership of their health and actively work towards positive outcomes.

II. Identifying Personal Priorities and Values:

Before setting goals, individuals with Type 2 diabetes must identify their personal priorities and values related to health and well-being. This involves reflecting on what matters most to them, their aspirations, and the areas of their life they wish to improve. By aligning health goals with personal values and priorities, individuals can enhance their motivation, commitment, and satisfaction with their efforts. For example, if spending quality time with family is a priority, setting goals related to managing diabetes to improve energy levels and overall health may be particularly meaningful.

III. Establishing Specific and Measurable Goals:

Effective goal setting involves establishing specific and measurable objectives that provide clarity and focus. Instead of setting vague goals such as "improve diabetes management," individuals should define precise targets that are observable and quantifiable. For example, a specific goal could be to achieve a target hemoglobin A1c (HbA1c) level of less than 7% within six months, as measured by regular blood tests. Measurable goals allow individuals to track their progress objectively and make adjustments to their action plan as needed.

IV. Setting Achievable and Realistic Goals:

It's essential to set goals that are achievable and realistic given one's circumstances, abilities, and resources. Unrealistic goals can lead to frustration, disappointment, and disengagement, undermining long-term success. When setting goals, individuals should consider factors such as their current health status, lifestyle preferences, available support networks, and potential barriers to success. Breaking larger goals into smaller, manageable steps can make them more attainable and increase confidence in one's ability to succeed.

V. Aligning Goals with Healthcare Recommendations:

Goal setting in Type 2 diabetes management should be aligned with healthcare recommendations and evidence-based guidelines. Healthcare professionals play a crucial role in helping individuals set appropriate goals based on their medical history, risk factors, and treatment plan. Collaborating with healthcare providers ensures that goals are realistic, safe, and tailored to individual needs. Healthcare professionals can provide guidance on setting goals related to blood sugar control, weight management, physical activity, medication adherence, and other aspects of diabetes self-care.

VI.   Tracking Progress and Celebrating Achievements:

Regularly monitoring progress towards established goals is essential for staying motivated and accountable. Individuals can use various methods to track their progress, such as keeping a journal, using mobile apps or wearable devices, or scheduling regular check-ins with healthcare providers. Celebrating achievements, no matter how small, reinforces positive behavior change and builds momentum towards long-term success. Recognizing progress boosts confidence and reinforces the belief that further goals are within reach.

VII.   Adjusting Goals as Needed:

Flexibility is key when it comes to goal setting, especially in managing Type 2 diabetes, where individual circumstances and health status may change over time. It's important to periodically review and reassess goals to ensure they remain relevant, achievable, and aligned with current needs and priorities. If circumstances or priorities shift, individuals may need to adjust their goals accordingly or set new objectives that better reflect their evolving situation. By remaining adaptable and responsive, individuals can maintain momentum and continue progressing towards improved health and well-being.

In conclusion, setting realistic goals is a foundational step in taking control of one's health, particularly for individuals with Type 2 diabetes. By establishing specific, measurable, achievable, and relevant goals that align with personal priorities and healthcare recommendations, individuals can create a roadmap for effectively managing their diabetes and improving their overall well-being. Through ongoing monitoring, adjustment, and celebration of achievements, individuals can stay motivated and empowered to make lasting changes that support their health and vitality.

3. Monitoring Blood Sugar Levels

Monitoring blood sugar levels is a crucial aspect of managing Type 2 diabetes and plays a significant role in maintaining optimal health and preventing complications. By regularly tracking blood glucose levels, individuals can gain valuable insights into how their bodies respond to various factors such as food, physical activity, medication, and stress. In this chapter, we explore the importance of monitoring blood sugar levels, different methods of monitoring, and practical tips for effective self-monitoring.

<h2 style="text-align:center">Importance of Monitoring Blood Sugar Levels:</h2>

Monitoring blood sugar levels is essential for individuals with Type 2 diabetes to assess their current glucose control, identify patterns and trends in blood sugar fluctuations, and make informed decisions about diabetes management. By monitoring regularly, individuals can detect hyperglycemia (high blood sugar) or hypoglycemia (low blood sugar) promptly and take appropriate action to prevent complications. Consistent monitoring also enables individuals to evaluate the effectiveness of their treatment plan, including medication, diet, exercise, and lifestyle modifications.

<h2 style="text-align:center">Methods of Monitoring Blood Sugar Levels:</h2>

There are several methods available for monitoring blood sugar levels, each with its advantages, limitations, and considerations. The primary methods include:

I. **Self-Monitoring of Blood Glucose (SMBG):** SMBG involves using a glucometer to measure blood sugar levels at home using a small drop of blood obtained from a finger prick. Glucometers provide immediate results and are convenient for regular monitoring throughout the day. They are suitable for individuals who require frequent blood sugar checks or have specific treatment goals, such as tight glucose control or insulin therapy.

II. **Continuous Glucose Monitoring (CGM):** CGM systems use sensors inserted under the skin to measure interstitial glucose levels continuously throughout the day and night. CGM devices provide real-time glucose readings, trend data, and alerts for high or low glucose levels. CGM is particularly useful for individuals who want more comprehensive glucose monitoring, including those on intensive insulin therapy or those with unpredictable glucose fluctuations.

III. **Hemoglobin A1c (HbA1c) Testing:** HbA1c testing measures the average blood sugar level over the past two to three months by assessing the percentage of glucose attached to hemoglobin in red blood cells. HbA1c testing provides an overall picture of long-term glucose control and is typically performed every three to six months as part of routine diabetes care. It complements SMBG and CGM by offering insight into glycemic trends over time.

Practical Tips for Effective Self-Monitoring:

To optimize blood sugar monitoring and derive maximum benefit from the process, individuals can follow these practical tips:

I.   **Establish a Monitoring Routine**: Develop a consistent schedule for monitoring blood sugar levels based on personal preferences, healthcare provider recommendations, and treatment goals. Regular monitoring helps maintain discipline and ensures that glucose levels are monitored at appropriate times throughout the day.

II.   **Keep Accurate Records**: Record blood sugar readings, along with relevant details such as the time of day, meals, physical activity, medication doses, and any symptoms experienced. Keeping accurate records allows individuals to track trends, identify patterns, and share information with healthcare providers for review and adjustment of treatment plans.

III.   **Pay Attention to Patterns and Trends**: Analyze blood sugar data regularly to identify patterns, trends, and factors that influence glucose levels. Look for recurring patterns such as postprandial spikes, overnight fluctuations, or exercise-related changes. Understanding these patterns can help individuals make targeted adjustments to their diabetes management strategies.

IV.   **Use Technology Wisely**: Leverage technology tools such as smartphone apps, digital platforms, and wearable devices to simplify blood sugar monitoring and data management. Many glucometers and CGM systems offer data-sharing capabilities, cloud storage, and analytics features to enhance monitoring efficiency and convenience.

V. Communicate with Healthcare Providers: Share blood sugar data and monitoring records with healthcare providers during regular appointments or consultations. Open communication ensures that healthcare providers have accurate and up-to-date information to assess glycemic control, identify areas for improvement, and make appropriate adjustments to treatment plans.

By incorporating these strategies into their diabetes management routine, individuals with Type 2 diabetes can take control of their health, optimize blood sugar control, and minimize the risk of complications. Monitoring blood sugar levels empowers individuals to make informed decisions about their diabetes care, leading to better health outcomes and an improved quality of life.

Chapter 4

Dietary Strategies for Managing Type 2 Diabetes.

1. Overview of Diabetes-Friendly Foods

In managing Type 2 diabetes, dietary strategies play a central role in controlling blood sugar levels, promoting weight management, and reducing the risk of complications. By adopting a balanced and diabetes-friendly eating plan, individuals can optimize their health and well-being while enjoying a variety of delicious and nutritious foods. In this chapter, we explore dietary strategies for managing Type 2 diabetes, with a focus on an overview of diabetes-friendly foods and practical tips for meal planning and preparation.

I. Understanding Diabetes-Friendly Foods:

Diabetes-friendly foods are those that help regulate blood sugar levels, provide essential nutrients, and support overall health. These foods are typically low in added sugars, saturated fats, and refined carbohydrates, while high in fiber, vitamins, minerals, and antioxidants. By choosing a variety of nutrient-dense foods, individuals with Type 2 diabetes can achieve better glycemic control, improve insulin sensitivity, and reduce the risk of cardiovascular disease.

- **Non-Starchy Vegetables**: Non-starchy vegetables are rich in fiber, vitamins, minerals, and antioxidants, making them an excellent choice for people with Type 2 diabetes. Examples include leafy greens (spinach, kale, lettuce), cruciferous vegetables (broccoli, cauliflower, Brussels sprouts), peppers, tomatoes, cucumbers, and zucchini. These vegetables have a low glycemic index, meaning they have minimal impact on blood sugar levels.
- **Lean Proteins**: Lean protein sources are essential for maintaining muscle mass, supporting satiety, and stabilizing blood sugar levels. Opt for lean cuts of meat such as skinless poultry, fish, seafood, and lean cuts of beef or pork. Other protein-rich options include tofu, tempeh, legumes (beans, lentils, chickpeas), eggs, and low-fat dairy products (Greek yogurt, cottage cheese).
- **Whole Grains**: Whole grains are rich in fiber, which helps slow down the absorption of glucose and prevents rapid spikes in blood sugar

levels. Choose whole grain options such as brown rice, quinoa, barley, oats, whole wheat bread, whole grain pasta, and bulgur. These grains provide sustained energy, promote satiety, and support digestive health.

- **Healthy Fats**: Healthy fats, such as monounsaturated and polyunsaturated fats, play a crucial role in heart health and insulin sensitivity. Include sources of healthy fats in your diet, such as avocado, nuts (almonds, walnuts, pistachios), seeds (chia seeds, flaxseeds, pumpkin seeds), olive oil, and fatty fish (salmon, mackerel, sardines). Limit saturated fats and avoid trans fats, which can increase the risk of cardiovascular disease.

- **Fruits:** While fruits contain natural sugars, they are also rich in fiber, vitamins, and antioxidants, making them a nutritious choice for people with Type 2 diabetes. Focus on whole fruits rather than fruit juices or dried fruits, which can be higher in sugar and lower in fiber. Opt for fresh or frozen fruits such as berries, apples, oranges, pears, and grapes, and limit portions to manage carbohydrate intake.

- **Dairy Alternatives**: For individuals who are lactose intolerant or prefer non-dairy options, there are various dairy alternatives available, including almond milk, soy milk, coconut milk, and oat milk. Choose unsweetened varieties to minimize added sugars and select fortified options to ensure adequate calcium and vitamin D intake.

II.   **Practical Tips for Meal Planning and Preparation:**

- **Prioritize Portion Control**: Pay attention to portion sizes and aim for balanced meals that include a combination of carbohydrates, protein, and healthy fats. Use measuring cups, food scales, or visual cues to estimate portion sizes and avoid overeating.

- **Choose Whole Foods:** Focus on whole, minimally processed foods whenever possible, as they tend to be lower in added sugars, sodium, and unhealthy fats. Incorporate a variety of colorful fruits, vegetables, whole grains, and lean proteins into your meals to maximize nutrient intake and flavor.

- **Experiment with Cooking Methods**: Explore different cooking techniques such as grilling, baking, steaming, sautéing, and roasting to enhance the flavor and texture of your meals without adding excess calories or unhealthy fats. Experiment with herbs, spices, and seasonings to add depth and complexity to your dishes.

- **Plan Ahead:** Take time to plan your meals and snacks for the week ahead, including grocery shopping and meal preparation. Batch cooking and meal prepping can save time and energy during busy weekdays and ensure that you have healthy options readily available when hunger strikes.

- **Practice Mindful Eating**: Be mindful of your eating habits, including hunger cues, satiety signals, and emotional triggers for eating. Slow down and savor each bite, chewing thoroughly and paying attention to taste, texture, and satisfaction. Avoid distractions such as TV, phones, or computers while eating to focus on the sensory experience of eating.

By incorporating these dietary strategies into your daily routine, you can take control of your health and effectively manage Type 2 diabetes. With a focus on diabetes-friendly foods, portion control, and mindful eating, you can enjoy delicious and nutritious meals while supporting your overall well-being and reducing the risk of complications.

2. Creating a Balanced Meal Plan.

Creating a balanced meal plan is essential for effectively managing Type 2 diabetes and optimizing overall health and well-being. By incorporating a variety of nutrient-dense foods and paying attention to portion sizes and macronutrient distribution, individuals with Type 2 diabetes can achieve better glycemic control, improve insulin sensitivity, and reduce the risk of complications. In this chapter, we explore dietary strategies for creating a balanced meal plan tailored to the needs of individuals with Type 2 diabetes.

I. Understanding Macronutrients:

Before creating a balanced meal plan, it's important to understand the role of macronutrients in the diet and how they affect blood sugar levels and overall health.

- **Carbohydrates:** Carbohydrates are the primary macronutrient that affects blood sugar levels. They are broken down into glucose, which is the body's main source of energy. While carbohydrates are an essential part of the diet, people with Type 2 diabetes need to be mindful of the types and amounts of carbohydrates they consume to prevent spikes in blood sugar levels. Focus on complex carbohydrates such as whole grains, fruits, vegetables, and legumes, which are rich in fiber and have a lower impact on blood sugar levels compared to refined carbohydrates.
- **Protein:** Protein plays a crucial role in building and repairing tissues, supporting immune function, and stabilizing blood sugar levels.

Include lean protein sources such as poultry, fish, tofu, legumes, and low-fat dairy products in your meals to promote satiety and maintain muscle mass. Aim to distribute protein intake evenly throughout the day to optimize muscle protein synthesis and blood sugar control.

- **Fat**: Dietary fat is an important source of energy and helps absorb fat-soluble vitamins, regulate hormones, and support cell function. Choose healthy fats such as monounsaturated and polyunsaturated fats found in nuts, seeds, avocado, olive oil, and fatty fish. Limit saturated fats and avoid trans fats, which can increase the risk of heart disease and insulin resistance.

- **Building a Balanced Plate:**

A balanced meal plan for managing Type 2 diabetes typically includes a combination of carbohydrates, protein, and healthy fats in appropriate portions. The plate method is a simple and effective tool for creating balanced meals and controlling portion sizes.

Fill Half Your Plate with Non-Starchy Vegetables: Non-starchy vegetables such as leafy greens, broccoli, cauliflower, peppers, and tomatoes are low in calories and carbohydrates but high in fiber, vitamins, and minerals. Fill half your plate with non-starchy vegetables to add volume and nutrients to your meals while keeping calories and carbohydrates in check.

Allocate One-Quarter of Your Plate to Lean Protein: Lean protein sources such as poultry, fish, tofu, legumes, and eggs should occupy one-quarter of your plate. Choose lean cuts of meat, remove visible fat, and opt for cooking methods that minimize added fats and oils.

Reserve One-Quarter of Your Plate for Whole Grains or Starchy Vegetables: Whole grains such as brown rice, quinoa, barley, oats, and whole grain bread should make up one-quarter of your plate. Alternatively, you can choose starchy vegetables such as sweet potatoes, corn, peas, or winter squash as a carbohydrate source. These foods provide energy and fiber while supporting blood sugar control.

Monitoring Portion Sizes:

In addition to balancing macronutrients, it's essential to pay attention to portion sizes to prevent overeating and manage blood sugar levels effectively. Use visual cues, measuring cups, or food scales to estimate portion sizes and avoid oversized servings.

Carbohydrates: A serving of carbohydrates is typically equivalent to 15 grams of carbohydrate. Examples of one carbohydrate serving include one slice of bread, 1/3 cup of cooked rice or pasta, or one small piece of fruit. Aim to include 45-60 grams of carbohydrates per meal, distributed evenly throughout the day.

Protein: A serving of protein is approximately 3-4 ounces, or about the size of a deck of cards. Include 15-30 grams of protein per meal to promote satiety and support muscle health.

Fat: While healthy fats are an important part of the diet, it's essential to monitor portion sizes to avoid excess calorie intake. Limit added fats and oils to 1-2 tablespoons per meal and choose unsaturated fats whenever possible.

Incorporating Snacks:

Snacks can help prevent blood sugar fluctuations between meals and provide additional nutrients and energy. Choose nutrient-dense snacks that combine carbohydrates, protein, and healthy fats to promote satiety and stabilize blood sugar levels. Examples of diabetes-friendly snacks include Greek yogurt with berries, apple slices with almond butter, raw vegetables with hummus, or a small handful of nuts and seeds.

By following these guidelines and creating a balanced meal plan, individuals with Type 2 diabetes can effectively manage their condition, optimize their health, and reduce the risk of complications. Consult with a registered dietitian or diabetes educator for personalized nutrition advice and support in developing a meal plan tailored to your individual needs and preferences.

3. Portion Control and Carb Counting

Portion control and carbohydrate counting are fundamental dietary strategies for managing Type 2 diabetes effectively. By understanding portion sizes and carbohydrate content in foods, individuals with diabetes can regulate blood sugar levels, maintain a healthy weight, and prevent complications. In this chapter, we delve into the principles of portion control and carb counting and provide practical tips for incorporating these strategies into daily life.

I.   Portion Control:

Portion control involves managing the amount of food consumed at each meal and snack to ensure a balanced intake of nutrients and prevent overeating. For individuals with Type 2 diabetes, portion control is particularly important to regulate blood sugar levels and achieve glycemic control.

- **Visual Cues:** Use visual cues to estimate portion sizes without relying on measuring cups or food scales. For example, a serving of meat should be about the size of a deck of cards, a serving of pasta or rice should be about the size of a tennis ball, and a serving of cheese should be about the size of a domino.
- **Plate Method:** The plate method is a simple and effective tool for portion control. Divide your plate into sections and fill half with non-starchy vegetables, one-quarter with lean protein, and one-quarter with carbohydrates. This approach ensures a balanced intake of nutrients and prevents overeating.
- **Mindful Eating:** Practice mindful eating by paying attention to hunger and fullness cues, eating slowly, and savoring each bite. Avoid distractions such as watching TV or using electronic devices while eating, as this can lead to mindless overeating.
- **Smaller Plates and Bowls:** Use smaller plates and bowls to control portion sizes and prevent overeating. Research suggests that people tend to eat less when they use smaller dinnerware, as it creates the illusion of larger portions.
- **Carbohydrate Counting:** Carbohydrate counting involves monitoring the amount of carbohydrates consumed at each meal and snack to manage blood sugar levels effectively. Since carbohydrates have the most significant impact on blood sugar, individuals with Type 2 diabetes need to be mindful of their carbohydrate intake and choose carbohydrate sources wisely.

II.   Identifying Carbohydrate Foods

Carbohydrate-containing foods include grains, starchy vegetables, fruits, dairy products, and sweets. Reading food labels and understanding food composition can help identify carbohydrate-containing foods and determine portion sizes.

Counting Carbohydrate Servings: Carbohydrates are typically measured in grams or servings. One serving of carbohydrates, also known as one carb choice, contains approximately 15 grams of carbohydrates. Aim to include a consistent amount of carbohydrates at each meal and snack to maintain stable blood sugar levels.

Planning Meals: Plan meals and snacks ahead of time to ensure a balanced intake of carbohydrates throughout the day. Use carbohydrate counting to determine appropriate portion sizes and adjust insulin or medication doses as needed to match carbohydrate intake.

Monitoring Blood Sugar Levels: Regularly monitor blood sugar levels to assess the impact of carbohydrate intake on glycemic control. Keep a log of carbohydrate intake, blood sugar readings, and medication doses to identify patterns and make adjustments as necessary.

Practical Tips:

Choose High-Fiber Carbohydrates: Opt for high-fiber carbohydrates such as whole grains, fruits, vegetables, and legumes, which have a lower glycemic index and provide sustained energy.

Be Mindful of Portion Sizes: Pay attention to portion sizes when consuming carbohydrate-containing foods, especially foods with added sugars or refined carbohydrates. Limit portion sizes of sweets, sugary beverages, and processed snacks to prevent blood sugar spikes.

Spread Carbohydrates Throughout the Day: Distribute carbohydrate intake evenly throughout the day to prevent large fluctuations in blood sugar levels. Avoid skipping meals or consuming large amounts of carbohydrates at once, as this can lead to unstable blood sugar levels.

By practicing portion control and carbohydrate counting, individuals with Type 2 diabetes can effectively manage their condition, achieve glycemic control, and improve overall health and well-being. Consult with a registered dietitian or diabetes educator for personalized nutrition advice and support in implementing these dietary strategies into your daily routine.

4. Managing Sugar and Sweeteners

Managing sugar and sweeteners is crucial for individuals with Type 2 diabetes to maintain stable blood sugar levels and prevent complications associated with the condition. While sugar and sweeteners can add flavor to foods and beverages, they can also contribute to elevated blood sugar levels if consumed in excess. In this chapter, we explore dietary strategies for managing sugar and sweeteners in the context of a diabetes-friendly meal plan.

I.   Understanding Sugar and Sweeteners:

Natural Sugars: Natural sugars are found naturally in foods such as fruits, vegetables, and dairy products. These sugars are accompanied by essential nutrients such as vitamins, minerals, and fiber, which can help regulate blood sugar levels. Examples of natural sugars include fructose (found in fruits) and lactose (found in dairy products).

Added Sugars: Added sugars are sugars that are added to foods and beverages during processing or preparation. These sugars provide empty calories and can contribute to weight gain and elevated blood sugar levels. Common sources of added sugars include sugary beverages, desserts, candies, and processed foods.

Artificial Sweeteners: Artificial sweeteners are sugar substitutes that provide sweetness without the calories or carbohydrates found in sugar. These sweeteners are often used in sugar-free or low-calorie products marketed to individuals with diabetes. Examples of artificial sweeteners include aspartame, sucralose, and saccharin.

II.   Tips for Managing Sugar and Sweeteners

Read Food Labels: Read food labels carefully to identify sources of added sugars in packaged foods and beverages. Look for terms such as sucrose, high-fructose corn syrup, and dextrose on the ingredient list, as these indicate the presence of added sugars.

Choose Whole Foods: Opt for whole foods such as fruits, vegetables, lean proteins, and whole grains, which are naturally low in added sugars and provide essential nutrients. Incorporate a variety of colorful fruits and vegetables into your meals and snacks to satisfy your sweet cravings while promoting overall health.

Limit Sugary Beverages: Limit consumption of sugary beverages such as sodas, fruit juices, and sweetened teas, as these can cause rapid spikes in blood sugar levels. Choose water, unsweetened tea, or sparkling water with a splash of lemon or lime for a refreshing and hydrating alternative.

Use Artificial Sweeteners Sparingly: Use artificial sweeteners in moderation as part of a balanced meal plan. While artificial sweeteners are low in calories and carbohydrates, some research suggests that excessive consumption may have adverse effects on metabolism and gut health. Stick to recommended serving sizes and consult with a healthcare professional if you have concerns about artificial sweeteners.

III.   Practical Tips for Sugar-Free Cooking and Baking:

Experiment with Natural Sweeteners: Experiment with natural sweeteners such as stevia, monk fruit extract, and erythritol as alternatives to sugar in cooking and baking. These sweeteners provide sweetness without affecting blood sugar levels and can be used in a variety of recipes.

Reduce Sugar in Recipes: Gradually reduce the amount of sugar called for in recipes to decrease the overall sugar content while still maintaining flavor. Substitute sugar with ingredients such as applesauce, mashed bananas, or Greek yogurt to add sweetness and moisture to baked goods.

Focus on Flavor: Enhance the flavor of dishes with herbs, spices, and citrus zest to reduce the need for added sugars. Incorporate ingredients such as cinnamon, vanilla, ginger, and nutmeg to add warmth and depth to dishes without relying on sugar for flavor.

By adopting these dietary strategies for managing sugar and sweeteners, individuals with Type 2 diabetes can enjoy delicious and satisfying meals while maintaining optimal blood sugar control. Experiment with different ingredients and cooking techniques to find what works best for you, and consult with a registered dietitian or diabetes educator for personalized nutrition advice and support.

Chapter 5
Incorporating Physical Activity into Your Routine

1. Benefits of Exercise for Diabetes Management

Incorporating physical activity into your routine is essential for managing Type 2 diabetes and promoting overall health and well-being. Regular exercise offers numerous benefits for individuals with diabetes, including improved blood sugar control, increased insulin sensitivity, weight management, and reduced risk of cardiovascular complications. In this chapter, we delve into the benefits of exercise for diabetes management and provide practical tips for incorporating physical activity into your daily life.

I. Improved Blood Sugar Control:

Regular physical activity helps to lower blood sugar levels by increasing the uptake of glucose by muscle cells, thereby reducing insulin resistance. Exercise stimulates the movement of glucose from the bloodstream into cells, where it can be used as energy. This process helps to regulate blood sugar levels and prevents spikes and crashes in glucose levels throughout the day.

II. Increased Insulin Sensitivity:

Exercise enhances insulin sensitivity, allowing the body to use insulin more effectively to regulate blood sugar levels. By engaging in regular physical activity, individuals with Type 2 diabetes can reduce their reliance on insulin medication and improve their overall metabolic health. Increased insulin sensitivity also helps to prevent the progression of insulin resistance, a hallmark of Type 2 diabetes.

III. Weight Management:

Regular exercise plays a crucial role in weight management and can help individuals with Type 2 diabetes achieve and maintain a healthy body weight. Physical activity helps to burn calories, build lean muscle mass, and boost metabolism, leading to improved body composition and weight loss. Maintaining a healthy weight is important for diabetes management as excess body fat can contribute to insulin resistance and worsen blood sugar control.

IV.   Cardiovascular Health:

Exercise has numerous cardiovascular benefits for individuals with Type 2 diabetes, including reduced risk of heart disease, stroke, and peripheral artery disease. Physical activity helps to strengthen the heart muscle, improve circulation, and lower blood pressure and cholesterol levels. Regular exercise also reduces inflammation and oxidative stress, which are known risk factors for cardiovascular complications in diabetes.

V.   Reduction and Mental Health:

Physical activity has been shown to reduce stress, anxiety, and depression, improving overall mental health and well-being. Engaging in regular exercise releases endorphins, neurotransmitters that promote feelings of happiness and relaxation. Exercise also provides an opportunity for social interaction and can help individuals with diabetes feel more connected to others and less isolated.

VI.   Practical Tips for Incorporating Exercise into Your Routine:

Start Slowly: If you're new to exercise or haven't been active for a while, start slowly and gradually increase the intensity and duration of your workouts. Aim for at least 150 minutes of moderate-intensity aerobic exercise per week, such as brisk walking, cycling, or swimming.

Find Activities You Enjoy: Choose activities that you enjoy and that fit into your lifestyle. Whether it's dancing, gardening, or playing a sport, finding enjoyable forms of exercise will make it easier to stick to a regular routine.

Make It a Habit: Schedule regular exercise sessions into your weekly routine and treat them like appointments that cannot be missed. Consistency is key to reaping the long-term benefits of exercise for diabetes management.

Mix It Up: Incorporate a variety of activities into your exercise routine to keep things interesting and prevent boredom. Try different types of workouts, such as strength training, yoga, or Pilates, to target different muscle groups and improve overall fitness.

By incorporating regular physical activity into your routine, you can improve blood sugar control, increase insulin sensitivity, manage your weight, and reduce your risk of cardiovascular complications. Make exercise a priority in

your diabetes management plan and enjoy the many benefits it has to offer for
your health and well-being.

2. Types of Exercise Suitable for Diabetics

Incorporating physical activity into your routine is crucial for managing Type
2 diabetes and promoting overall health. When it comes to exercise, there are
various types that are suitable for individuals with diabetes, each offering
unique benefits for blood sugar control, cardiovascular health, and overall
well-being. In this chapter, we explore different types of exercise that are
suitable for diabetics and provide practical tips for incorporating them into
your routine.

I.   Aerobic Exercise:

Aerobic exercise, also known as cardio or endurance exercise, involves
repetitive movements that increase your heart rate and breathing. This type of
exercise is particularly beneficial for improving cardiovascular health, burning
calories, and lowering blood sugar levels. Examples of aerobic exercises
suitable for diabetics include:

II.   Walking:

 Walking is one of the most accessible and convenient forms of aerobic
exercise. It can be done virtually anywhere, requires no special equipment, and
can be easily modified to suit your fitness level. Aim for brisk walking sessions
of at least 30 minutes most days of the week to reap the benefits for blood
sugar control and cardiovascular health.

III.   Cycling:

Cycling is another low-impact aerobic exercise that is gentle on the joints and
provides a great cardiovascular workout. Whether you prefer riding outdoors
or using a stationary bike indoors, cycling can help improve endurance,
strengthen leg muscles, and enhance overall fitness.

IV.   Swimming:

 Swimming is an excellent full-body workout that is easy on the joints and
suitable for individuals of all fitness levels. It provides resistance training for
muscle strength and endurance while also improving cardiovascular fitness
and flexibility. Swimming laps or participating in water aerobics classes can be
an enjoyable way to stay active and manage diabetes.

V.   Strength Training:

Strength training, also known as resistance training or weightlifting, involves using resistance to build muscle strength, endurance, and power. While aerobic exercise primarily targets the cardiovascular system, strength training focuses on building and toning muscles, which can have numerous benefits for individuals with diabetes. Examples of strength training exercises suitable for diabetics include:

VI.   Bodyweight Exercises:

Bodyweight exercises, such as squats, lunges, push-ups, and planks, use your own body weight as resistance to build strength and muscle tone. These exercises can be performed at home or in the gym with minimal equipment and are suitable for beginners and advanced exercisers alike.

Resistance Bands: Resistance bands are lightweight, portable, and versatile tools that can be used to perform a wide range of strength training exercises. They provide variable resistance, allowing you to adjust the intensity of your workouts to suit your fitness level. Resistance band exercises can target specific muscle groups and help improve overall strength and stability.

VII.   Free Weights:

Free weights, such as dumbbells, kettlebells, and barbells, offer a more traditional form of strength training that allows for greater resistance and progression over time. Incorporating free weight exercises into your routine can help increase muscle mass, improve bone density, and enhance metabolic health.

VIII.   Flexibility and Balance Exercises:

Flexibility and balance exercises are often overlooked but are essential components of a well-rounded exercise routine, especially for individuals with diabetes. These types of exercises help improve joint mobility, range of motion, and proprioception, reducing the risk of falls and injuries. Examples of flexibility and balance exercises suitable for diabetics include:

IX.   Yoga:

Yoga is a gentle form of exercise that combines stretching, breathing, and meditation to improve flexibility, balance, and relaxation. Practicing yoga regularly can help reduce stress, lower blood pressure, and improve overall mental and physical well-being. There are various styles of yoga to choose from, ranging from gentle restorative practices to more dynamic vinyasa flows.

X.   Tai Chi:

Tai Chi is a low-impact mind-body exercise that originated in ancient China and is often referred to as "meditation in motion." It involves slow, flowing movements performed in a relaxed and mindful manner, promoting balance, coordination, and stress reduction. Tai Chi has been shown to improve balance, reduce falls, and enhance overall quality of life for individuals with diabetes.

XI.   Stretching:

Stretching exercises help improve flexibility, reduce muscle tension, and prevent injury by lengthening tight muscles and improving joint mobility. Incorporating stretching into your routine can help alleviate stiffness, improve posture, and enhance overall movement quality. Focus on stretching major muscle groups, such as the calves, hamstrings, quadriceps, chest, shoulders, and back, holding each stretch for 15-30 seconds and repeating 2-3 times.

Incorporating a variety of exercises into your routine, including aerobic, strength training, flexibility, and balance exercises, can help you achieve optimal health and well-being while managing Type 2 diabetes. Aim for a balanced exercise program that includes a mix of different activities to target different aspects of fitness and enjoy the numerous benefits that regular physical activity has to offer.

3. Developing an Exercise Plan.

Developing an exercise plan is essential for incorporating physical activity into your routine and effectively managing Type 2 diabetes. A well-thought-out plan can help you set realistic goals, stay motivated, and establish a consistent exercise routine that fits your lifestyle and preferences. In this chapter, we will discuss the key components of developing an exercise plan for individuals with diabetes and provide practical tips for creating a personalized approach to physical activity.

I.   Assess Your Current Fitness Level:

Before embarking on an exercise plan, it's important to assess your current fitness level to determine your baseline capabilities and identify any limitations or health concerns. Consider factors such as your age, overall health, fitness history, and any existing medical conditions that may impact your ability to exercise safely. Consulting with your healthcare provider or a qualified exercise professional can help you assess your fitness level and develop a tailored plan that meets your needs.

II.   Set Realistic Goals:

Setting realistic and achievable goals is crucial for staying motivated and making progress with your exercise plan. Start by identifying specific objectives that align with your overall health and fitness goals, such as improving blood sugar control, losing weight, increasing muscle strength, or enhancing cardiovascular endurance. Break down your goals into smaller, manageable steps and establish a timeline for achieving them. Consider using the SMART criteria (Specific, Measurable, Achievable, Relevant, Time-bound) to ensure that your goals are well-defined and actionable.

III.   Choose Activities You Enjoy:

One of the keys to sticking with an exercise plan is selecting activities that you enjoy and find enjoyable. Experiment with different types of exercises, such as walking, cycling, swimming, yoga, strength training, or group fitness classes, to discover what works best for you. Consider your preferences, interests, and lifestyle factors when choosing activities and aim to incorporate a variety of exercises into your routine to keep it interesting and engaging.

IV.   Gradually Increase Intensity and Duration:

When starting an exercise program, it's important to start slowly and gradually increase the intensity, duration, and frequency of your workouts over time. Begin with low-impact activities at a comfortable intensity level and gradually progress as your fitness improves. Aim for at least 150 minutes of moderate-intensity aerobic exercise or 75 minutes of vigorous-intensity aerobic exercise per week, spread out over several days, along with two or more days of strength training exercises targeting major muscle groups.

V.   Incorporate Physical Activity into Your Daily Routine:

Finding opportunities to be physically active throughout the day can help you meet your exercise goals and maintain a consistent routine. Look for ways to incorporate movement into your daily activities, such as taking the stairs instead of the elevator, parking farther away from your destination, walking or biking to work, gardening, dancing, or playing active games with family and friends. Breaking up sedentary time with short bursts of activity can help improve blood sugar control and reduce the risk of complications associated with prolonged sitting.

VI.   Listen to Your Body and Adapt as Needed:

Listen to your body and pay attention to how you feel during and after exercise. If you experience pain, discomfort, dizziness, or other symptoms, stop exercising immediately and seek medical attention if necessary. Be flexible and willing to adapt your exercise plan based on your changing needs, preferences, and circumstances. Modify your workouts as needed to accommodate any health concerns or physical limitations, and don't hesitate to seek guidance from a healthcare professional or certified fitness trainer if you have questions or need support.

By following these guidelines and developing a personalized exercise plan that aligns with your goals, preferences, and abilities, you can effectively incorporate physical activity into your routine and take control of your health while managing Type 2 diabetes. Remember to stay consistent, stay motivated, and celebrate your progress along the way as you work towards achieving your health and fitness goals.

chapter 6

Lifestyle Changes for Better Diabetes Management

1. Stress Management Techniques

Stress management is a crucial component of effective diabetes management, as chronic stress can negatively impact blood sugar levels and exacerbate symptoms of Type 2 diabetes. Learning how to cope with stress and implementing stress management techniques can help you reduce the harmful effects of stress on your body and improve your overall well-being. In this chapter, we will explore various stress management strategies that can help you better manage your diabetes and lead a healthier lifestyle.

I. Identify Sources of Stress:

The first step in managing stress is to identify the sources or triggers of stress in your life. Take some time to reflect on the factors that contribute to your stress levels, such as work, relationships, financial concerns, health issues, or daily hassles. Keep a journal or use a stress-tracking app to record stressful events and how they affect your mood, energy levels, and physical symptoms. By pinpointing the specific stressors in your life, you can develop targeted strategies for managing them more effectively.

II. Practice Relaxation Techniques:

Relaxation techniques are powerful tools for reducing stress and promoting relaxation in both mind and body. Incorporating relaxation exercises into your daily routine can help you unwind, relieve tension, and alleviate symptoms of stress. Experiment with different techniques such as deep breathing exercises, progressive muscle relaxation, guided imagery, meditation, yoga, tai chi, or mindfulness meditation. Find a method that resonates with you and practice it regularly to reap the benefits of relaxation.

III. Engage in Physical Activity:

Regular physical activity is not only beneficial for managing diabetes but also for reducing stress levels and improving mood. Exercise releases endorphins, the body's natural stress-relieving hormones, which can help you feel more relaxed and energized. Aim for at least 30 minutes of moderate-intensity aerobic exercise most days of the week, such as walking, jogging, cycling, swimming, or dancing. Incorporate strength training exercises into your routine to build muscle strength and improve overall fitness.

IV.   Prioritize Self-Care:

Taking care of yourself is essential for managing stress and maintaining your physical and emotional well-being. Make self-care a priority by carving out time for activities that nourish your body, mind, and soul. Practice good sleep hygiene by establishing a regular sleep schedule, creating a relaxing bedtime routine, and ensuring a comfortable sleep environment. Eat a balanced diet rich in nutritious foods that support optimal health and energy levels. Make time for hobbies, interests, and activities that bring you joy and fulfillment.

V.   Build a Strong Support Network:

Having a strong support network of friends, family members, healthcare professionals, and peers who understand and empathize with your experiences can provide invaluable emotional support during times of stress. Reach out to trusted individuals in your life for encouragement, guidance, and companionship. Join a diabetes support group or online community where you can connect with others who share similar challenges and experiences. Sharing your feelings and experiences with others who understand can help you feel less isolated and more supported in your diabetes journey.

VI.   Seek Professional Help When Needed:

If you find that stress is significantly impacting your quality of life or ability to manage your diabetes effectively, don't hesitate to seek professional help. A mental health counselor, therapist, or psychologist can provide you with strategies and coping skills to better manage stress and improve your emotional resilience. Your healthcare provider may also be able to recommend resources or refer you to specialized diabetes counseling services or stress management programs in your area.

Incorporating stress management techniques into your daily routine can help you better cope with the challenges of living with Type 2 diabetes and lead a healthier, more balanced life. Experiment with different strategies, be patient with yourself, and give yourself permission to prioritize your mental and emotional well-being. By taking proactive steps to manage stress, you can improve your diabetes management outcomes and enhance your overall quality of life.

2. Improving Sleep Quality

Improving sleep quality is paramount for effective diabetes management, as it directly impacts blood sugar levels, overall health, and quality of life. In this chapter, we will delve into the significance of sleep quality for individuals with diabetes and explore actionable strategies to enhance sleep hygiene and promote restful sleep.

I. Understanding the Importance of Sleep Quality:

Quality sleep is essential for regulating glucose metabolism, insulin sensitivity, and hormone production, all of which play crucial roles in diabetes management. Poor sleep quality or insufficient sleep can disrupt these processes, leading to elevated blood sugar levels, insulin resistance, weight gain, and increased risk of diabetes complications. Moreover, inadequate sleep can contribute to fatigue, mood disturbances, cognitive impairment, and compromised immune function, further exacerbating diabetes-related challenges.

II. Identifying Factors Affecting Sleep Quality:

Several factors can influence sleep quality in individuals with diabetes, including fluctuations in blood sugar levels, medications, coexisting sleep disorders (such as sleep apnea or restless leg syndrome), lifestyle habits, stress, and environmental factors. Understanding these factors is crucial for implementing targeted interventions to improve sleep quality and enhance overall well-being.

III. Implementing Sleep Hygiene Practices:

Establishing healthy sleep hygiene practices can significantly improve sleep quality and support diabetes management. These practices include:

Consistency: Maintaining a consistent sleep schedule by going to bed and waking up at the same time every day, even on weekends.

Environment: Creating a conducive sleep environment that is cool, dark, quiet, and comfortable, free from distractions such as electronic devices.

Relaxation Techniques: Incorporating relaxation techniques such as deep breathing, meditation, or progressive muscle relaxation to promote relaxation and reduce stress before bedtime.

Limiting Stimulants: Avoiding stimulants such as caffeine, nicotine, and alcohol close to bedtime, as they can interfere with sleep onset and quality.

Bedtime Routine: Establishing a relaxing bedtime routine to signal to the body that it is time to wind down, which may include activities such as reading, taking a warm bath, or practicing gentle yoga.

Managing Stress: Implementing stress management strategies such as mindfulness, journaling, or engaging in calming activities to alleviate stress and promote relaxation.

IV. Addressing Underlying Sleep Disorders:

For individuals experiencing persistent sleep disturbances, it is essential to identify and address any underlying sleep disorders. Consultation with a healthcare provider or sleep specialist may be necessary to evaluate symptoms, conduct sleep studies if indicated, and develop a tailored treatment plan. Treatments for sleep disorders may include continuous positive airway pressure (CPAP) therapy for sleep apnea, medication for insomnia, or lifestyle modifications.

V. Prioritizing Sleep as a Component of Diabetes Management:

Recognizing the integral role of sleep in diabetes management, individuals should prioritize sleep as part of their overall diabetes care routine. By adopting healthy sleep habits and making sleep a priority, individuals can optimize their health outcomes, better regulate blood sugar levels, and enhance their quality of life.

3. Smoking Cessation Strategies

In this chapter, we will explore the importance of smoking cessation for individuals with diabetes and discuss effective strategies to support smoking cessation efforts as part of a comprehensive approach to diabetes management.

I. Understanding the Link Between Smoking and Diabetes:

Smoking is a well-established risk factor for the development and progression of type 2 diabetes. It is associated with insulin resistance, impaired glucose metabolism, inflammation, and endothelial dysfunction, all of which contribute to the pathophysiology of diabetes. Additionally, smoking increases the risk of diabetes-related complications such as cardiovascular disease, neuropathy, nephropathy, and retinopathy. Therefore, quitting smoking is essential for improving overall health and reducing the burden of diabetes-related complications.

## II.	Benefits of Smoking Cessation for Diabetes Management:

Quitting smoking offers numerous benefits for individuals with diabetes, including:

Improved Glycemic Control: Smoking cessation has been shown to improve insulin sensitivity and reduce blood sugar levels, leading to better glycemic control.

Reduced Risk of Complications: By quitting smoking, individuals can lower their risk of developing diabetes-related complications, such as cardiovascular disease, neuropathy, and kidney disease.

Enhanced Cardiovascular Health: Smoking cessation lowers the risk of cardiovascular events such as heart attack, stroke, and peripheral artery disease, which are major causes of morbidity and mortality in individuals with diabetes.

Improved Respiratory Function: Quitting smoking can improve lung function and reduce the risk of respiratory infections, benefiting overall respiratory health.

## III.	Effective Smoking Cessation Strategies:

Several evidence-based strategies can support individuals with diabetes in their efforts to quit smoking:

Behavioral Counseling: Counseling and support from healthcare providers, counselors, or smoking cessation specialists can help individuals develop coping strategies, set goals, and navigate challenges associated with quitting smoking.

Nicotine Replacement Therapy (NRT): NRT products such as nicotine patches, gum, lozenges, and inhalers can help alleviate nicotine withdrawal symptoms and cravings, making it easier to quit smoking.

Prescription Medications: Certain prescription medications, such as bupropion (Zyban) and varenicline (Chantix), can aid in smoking cessation by reducing cravings and withdrawal symptoms.

Support Groups: Participating in support groups or smoking cessation programs can provide encouragement, accountability, and peer support for individuals attempting to quit smoking.

Stress Management: Developing alternative stress management techniques such as exercise, mindfulness, or relaxation exercises can help individuals cope with stress without resorting to smoking.

Lifestyle Modification: Encouraging lifestyle changes such as regular physical activity, healthy eating habits, and adequate sleep can complement smoking cessation efforts and promote overall well-being.

IV.   Incorporating Smoking Cessation into Diabetes Care:

Healthcare providers play a crucial role in supporting smoking cessation among individuals with diabetes. They can offer counscling, prescribe cessation medications, refer to specialized cessation programs, and provide ongoing monitoring and support to help patients quit smoking successfully. Additionally, integrating smoking cessation interventions into routine diabetes care can enhance overall diabetes management and improve long-term health outcomes.

In conclusion, smoking cessation is an essential component of comprehensive diabetes management, offering significant health benefits and reducing the risk of diabetes-related complications. By implementing evidence-based smoking cessation strategies and receiving support from healthcare providers, individuals with diabetes can successfully quit smoking and improve their overall health and well-being.

Chapter 7

Medication Management and Treatment Options.

1. Overview of Common Diabetes Medications

In this chapter, we will provide an overview of the common medications used in the management of diabetes, including their mechanisms of action, indications, and potential side effects.

I.   Metformin:

Mechanism of Action

 Metformin is a first-line oral medication for type 2 diabetes that works by reducing hepatic glucose production, increasing insulin sensitivity in peripheral tissues, and decreasing intestinal glucose absorption.

Indications: Metformin is indicated for the treatment of type 2 diabetes, particularly in overweight and obese individuals, and is often prescribed as initial therapy or in combination with other antidiabetic agents.

Side Effects: Common side effects of metformin include gastrointestinal symptoms such as nausea, vomiting, diarrhea, and abdominal discomfort. Rare but serious side effects may include lactic acidosis, particularly in individuals with renal impairment.

II.   Sulfonylureas:

Mechanism of Action

 Sulfonylureas stimulate insulin secretion from pancreatic beta cells by binding to sulfonylurea receptors on the beta cell membrane and closing ATP-sensitive potassium channels, leading to depolarization and calcium influx.

Indications: Sulfonylureas are used to lower blood sugar levels in individuals with type 2 diabetes who have adequate pancreatic beta cell function and are not responsive to lifestyle modifications or metformin therapy.

Side Effects: Common side effects of sulfonylureas include hypoglycemia, weight gain, and gastrointestinal upset. Rare but serious side effects may include allergic reactions, hematologic abnormalities, and liver toxicity.

III.   DPP-4 Inhibitors

Mechanism of Action

Dipeptidyl peptidase-4 (DPP-4) inhibitors increase insulin secretion and decrease glucagon secretion by inhibiting the enzymatic degradation of incretin hormones such as glucagon-like peptide-1 (GLP-1) and glucose-dependent insulinotropic peptide (GIP).

Indications: DPP-4 inhibitors are indicated for the treatment of type 2 diabetes as monotherapy or in combination with other antidiabetic agents, including metformin, sulfonylureas, and insulin.

Side Effects: Common side effects of DPP-4 inhibitors include upper respiratory tract infections, headache, nasopharyngitis, and gastrointestinal symptoms. Rare but serious side effects may include pancreatitis, hypersensitivity reactions, and joint pain.

IV.   GLP-1 Receptor Agonists:

Mechanism of Action

GLP-1 receptor agonists mimic the action of endogenous GLP-1 hormones by stimulating insulin secretion, inhibiting glucagon secretion, slowing gastric emptying, and promoting satiety.

Indications: GLP-1 receptor agonists are used for the treatment of type 2 diabetes to improve glycemic control and promote weight loss. They are available as injectable formulations for once-daily or once-weekly administration.

Side Effects: Common side effects of GLP-1 receptor agonists include nausea, vomiting, diarrhea, and injection site reactions. Rare but serious side effects may include pancreatitis, thyroid cancer, and acute kidney injury.

V.   Insulin:

Mechanism of Action

Insulin is a hormone that regulates blood sugar levels by promoting glucose uptake into cells, inhibiting hepatic glucose production, and stimulating glycogen synthesis.

Indications: Insulin therapy is indicated for individuals with type 1 diabetes who have absolute insulin deficiency and for those with type 2 diabetes who require insulin supplementation due to inadequate glycemic control despite oral antidiabetic agents.

Side Effects: Common side effects of insulin therapy include hypoglycemia, weight gain, injection site reactions, and allergic reactions. Individualized insulin regimens and careful monitoring are essential to minimize the risk of hypoglycemia and optimize glycemic control.

Overall, understanding the mechanisms of action, indications, and side effects of common diabetes medications is essential for healthcare providers and individuals with diabetes to make informed treatment decisions and achieve optimal glycemic control while minimizing the risk of adverse effects.

In conclusion, improving sleep quality is a crucial aspect of diabetes management that requires attention and proactive intervention. By implementing evidence-based sleep hygiene practices, addressing underlying sleep disorders, and prioritizing sleep as part of diabetes care, individuals can enhance their overall well-being and achieve better diabetes outcomes.

2. **Insulin Therapy**

   In this chapter, we will delve into insulin therapy as a crucial aspect of medication management and treatment options for individuals with diabetes. Insulin therapy plays a pivotal role in managing both type 1 and type 2 diabetes by regulating blood sugar levels and preventing complications associated with hyperglycemia.

Types of Insulin:

I. **Rapid-acting insulin**

Rapid-acting insulin analogs such as insulin lispro, insulin aspart, and insulin glulisine have a quick onset of action (within 15 minutes), peak in 1 to 2 hours, and last for 3 to 4 hours. They are typically administered just before meals to control postprandial glucose levels.

II.   Short-acting insulin

Regular human insulin has a slower onset of action (30 to 60 minutes), peaks in 2 to 3 hours, and lasts for 6 to 8 hours. It is commonly used to cover mealtime glucose spikes or as part of a basal-bolus insulin regimen.

III.   Intermediate-acting insulin

Intermediate-acting insulins such as NPH insulin have a delayed onset of action (1 to 2 hours), peak in 4 to 8 hours, and last for 12 to 16 hours. They provide basal insulin coverage and are often combined with rapid-acting or short-acting insulins to mimic physiological insulin secretion.

IV.   Long-acting insulin

Long-acting insulin analogs such as insulin glargine and insulin detemir have a prolonged duration of action (up to 24 hours) with relatively constant blood levels, providing basal insulin coverage throughout the day and night.

Insulin Administration:

I.   Subcutaneous injection

Insulin is typically administered subcutaneously into the fatty tissue of the abdomen, thigh, or upper arm using insulin syringes, pen devices, or insulin pumps. Injection sites should be rotated to prevent lipohypertrophy and ensure consistent insulin absorption.

II.   Insulin pump therapy

Insulin pumps deliver rapid-acting insulin continuously through a subcutaneous catheter, allowing for precise insulin dosing and flexibility in mealtime boluses. Pump therapy requires regular blood glucose monitoring and adjustment of insulin settings by the user or healthcare provider.

III.   Insulin Regimen:

Basal-bolus regimen: This regimen combines a long-acting or intermediate-acting insulin (basal insulin) to provide continuous background insulin coverage with rapid-acting or short-acting insulin (bolus insulin) to cover meals and correct hyperglycemia.

Fixed-dose insulin regimen: In this regimen, a fixed dose of insulin is administered at predetermined times throughout the day, regardless of meal intake. It is often used in individuals with type 2 diabetes who require insulin supplementation but have a predictable meal pattern.

Insulin intensification: Insulin therapy may need to be intensified over time to achieve glycemic targets and prevent complications. This may involve increasing insulin doses, adding or switching insulin formulations, or incorporating additional medications such as GLP-1 receptor agonists.

Monitoring and Adjusting Insulin Therapy:

Blood glucose monitoring: Regular self-monitoring of blood glucose levels is essential for adjusting insulin doses, assessing treatment efficacy, and preventing hypoglycemia and hyperglycemia.

Insulin dose adjustment: Insulin doses should be individualized based on factors such as carbohydrate intake, physical activity, illness, stress, and changes in weight or insulin sensitivity. Healthcare providers may use insulin-to-carbohydrate ratios, correction factors, and insulin sensitivity factors to guide dose adjustments.

Overall, insulin therapy is a cornerstone of diabetes management, offering individuals with diabetes the flexibility and control to optimize their blood sugar levels and improve their quality of life. Understanding the various types of insulin, administration techniques, regimens, and monitoring strategies is essential for successful insulin therapy and achieving glycemic targets.

3.   Alternative and Complementary Therapies

In this chapter, we explore alternative and complementary therapies as part of medication management and treatment options for individuals with diabetes. While conventional medications like insulin and oral antidiabetic drugs are widely used, there is growing interest in complementary approaches to complement traditional diabetes management strategies.

I.   Dietary Supplements:

Chromium: Chromium is a mineral that plays a role in insulin action and glucose metabolism. Some studies suggest that chromium supplementation may improve insulin sensitivity and lower blood sugar levels in individuals with diabetes. However, the evidence is mixed, and more research is needed to confirm its effectiveness.

Alpha-lipoic acid: Alpha-lipoic acid is an antioxidant that has been studied for its potential benefits in diabetes management. It may help improve insulin sensitivity, reduce oxidative stress, and alleviate neuropathic symptoms associated with diabetes. However, more research is needed to establish its efficacy and optimal dosage.

Cinnamon: Cinnamon is a spice that has been investigated for its potential antidiabetic properties. Some studies suggest that cinnamon supplementation may lower fasting blood sugar levels and improve insulin sensitivity in individuals with type 2 diabetes. However, the evidence is inconclusive, and further research is warranted.

Berberine: Berberine is a compound found in several plants, including goldenseal and barberry. It has been studied for its potential antidiabetic effects, such as improving insulin sensitivity, reducing glucose production in the liver, and lowering blood sugar levels. Preliminary research suggests that berberine supplementation may be beneficial for individuals with type 2 diabetes, but more high-quality studies are needed to confirm its efficacy and safety.

Herbal Remedies:

Gymnema sylvestre: Gymnema sylvestre is a traditional herb used in Ayurvedic medicine for its purported antidiabetic properties. It may help lower blood sugar levels by blocking sugar absorption in the intestines and stimulating insulin secretion from the pancreas. Some studies suggest that gymnema supplementation may improve glycemic control in individuals with type 2 diabetes, but more research is needed.

Bitter melon: Bitter melon, also known as bitter gourd or Momordica charantia, is a vegetable commonly consumed in Asian cuisines. It contains compounds that may have hypoglycemic effects, such as charantin, vicine, and polypeptide-p. Some studies suggest that bitter melon supplementation may help lower blood sugar levels and improve insulin sensitivity in individuals with diabetes. However, more research is needed to confirm its efficacy and safety.

Mind-Body Practices:

Yoga: Yoga is a mind-body practice that combines physical postures, breathing exercises, and meditation techniques. It has been studied for its potential benefits in diabetes management, such as improving glycemic control, reducing stress, and enhancing overall well-being. Some research suggests that regular yoga practice may help lower blood sugar levels and improve insulin sensitivity in individuals with type 2 diabetes.

Meditation: Meditation involves focusing the mind and achieving a state of deep relaxation and inner peace. It has been studied for its potential effects on stress reduction, emotional well-being, and glycemic control in individuals with diabetes. Some studies suggest that meditation techniques such as mindfulness meditation may help lower blood sugar levels and improve insulin sensitivity.

Acupuncture:

Acupuncture is a traditional Chinese medicine practice that involves inserting thin needles into specific points on the body to stimulate energy flow and promote healing. It has been studied for its potential effects on pain relief, stress reduction, and glycemic control in individuals with diabetes. Some research suggests that acupuncture may help improve insulin sensitivity, reduce diabetes-related complications, and enhance overall quality of life.

While alternative and complementary therapies may offer additional options for individuals with diabetes, it is essential to consult with a healthcare provider before incorporating them into your treatment plan. Some supplements and herbal remedies may interact with medications or have adverse effects, particularly in individuals with underlying health conditions. Additionally, more research is needed to establish the safety, efficacy, and optimal dosage of these therapies for diabetes management.

Chapter 8

Overcoming Challenges and Staying Motivated.

1. Dealing with Diabetes Burnout

In this chapter, we delve into the topic of dealing with diabetes burnout, a common challenge faced by individuals managing type 2 diabetes. Diabetes burnout refers to feelings of frustration, exhaustion, and apathy that can arise from the constant demands of diabetes self-care and management. It can manifest as a reluctance to adhere to treatment plans, monitor blood sugar levels, or engage in healthy behaviors, leading to suboptimal diabetes control and increased risk of complications.

I.   Recognizing the Signs of Diabetes Burnout

Diabetes burnout can manifest in various ways, including feelings of overwhelm, resentment towards diabetes management tasks, avoidance of healthcare appointments, neglecting self-care practices, and fluctuations in blood sugar levels. It is essential for individuals with diabetes and their healthcare providers to recognize the signs of burnout early to address them effectively.

II.   Understanding the Causes of Diabetes Burnout:

Several factors can contribute to diabetes burnout, including the chronic nature of the condition, the daily demands of diabetes management, fear of complications, unrealistic expectations, social stigma, and psychological factors such as depression, anxiety, and stress. Additionally, life events such as job loss, relationship issues, financial stress, or other health problems can exacerbate feelings of burnout.

III.   Coping Strategies for Diabetes Burnout:

Acknowledge and Accept Feelings: It's important for individuals with diabetes to acknowledge and accept their feelings of burnout without judgment. Denying or suppressing these emotions can intensify stress and lead to further disengagement from diabetes management.

Seek Support: Building a support network of family, friends, healthcare professionals, and peers who understand the challenges of living with diabetes can provide invaluable emotional support and practical assistance. Joining diabetes support groups, online forums, or attending counseling sessions can also offer opportunities to connect with others facing similar struggles.

Set Realistic Goals: Break down diabetes management tasks into manageable steps and set realistic goals that align with your capabilities and priorities. Celebrate small victories along the way and focus on progress rather than perfection.

Practice Self-Compassion: Be kind and compassionate towards yourself, especially during difficult times. Recognize that managing diabetes is a continuous journey with ups and downs, and it's okay to seek help when needed.

Take Breaks and Engage in Self-Care: Prioritize self-care activities that promote relaxation, stress reduction, and overall well-being. Engage in hobbies, exercise, mindfulness practices, or spend time with loved ones to recharge and rejuvenate.

Explore Treatment Options: If feelings of burnout persist despite self-care efforts, consider seeking professional help from a healthcare provider, therapist, or counselor who specializes in diabetes management and mental health. They can offer personalized guidance, coping strategies, and treatment options to address underlying issues contributing to burnout.

By acknowledging the challenges of diabetes burnout and implementing effective coping strategies, individuals can overcome feelings of overwhelm and regain motivation to effectively manage their diabetes and lead a fulfilling life. Remember that seeking support is a sign of strength, and you are not alone in your journey towards better diabetes management and overall well-being.

2.   Handling Social and Emotional Aspects

In this chapter, we explore the social and emotional aspects of managing type 2 diabetes and provide practical strategies for handling these challenges while staying motivated in your diabetes management journey.

I.   Navigating Social Situations:

Managing diabetes often involves navigating social situations where food choices, alcohol consumption, and meal timings may be different from your usual routine. It's essential to communicate your dietary needs and preferences assertively with friends, family, and coworkers to ensure that social gatherings accommodate your diabetes management plan.

Educate Others: Take the opportunity to educate those around you about diabetes and its management. By raising awareness and dispelling misconceptions, you can foster understanding and support from your social circle.

II.   Coping with Emotional Distress:

Living with a chronic condition like diabetes can take a toll on your emotional well-being. It's natural to experience a range of emotions, including frustration, anger, fear, sadness, or anxiety, at different stages of your diabetes journey. Acknowledge and validate your feelings while seeking healthy ways to cope with them.

Practice Mindfulness: Mindfulness techniques, such as deep breathing, meditation, or yoga, can help reduce stress, improve emotional resilience, and enhance overall well-being. Incorporate mindfulness practices into your daily routine to cultivate a greater sense of calm and balance.

Seek Emotional Support: Don't hesitate to reach out for emotional support from trusted friends, family members, support groups, or mental health professionals. Sharing your feelings and experiences with others who understand can provide comfort, validation, and encouragement.

III.   Building Resilience:

Cultivate resilience by adopting a positive mindset and reframing challenges as opportunities for growth and learning. Focus on your strengths, accomplishments, and past successes in managing diabetes, and draw inspiration from them during difficult times.

Set Realistic Expectations: Accept that living with diabetes may involve setbacks and challenges along the way. Set realistic expectations for yourself and celebrate progress, no matter how small. Remember that every step forward counts towards your overall health and well-being.

Celebrate Achievements: Acknowledge and celebrate your achievements and milestones in diabetes management, whether it's reaching a target blood sugar level, adhering to your medication regimen, or making positive lifestyle changes. Reward yourself for your efforts and recognize the hard work you've put in.

By addressing the social and emotional aspects of diabetes management and implementing effective coping strategies, you can navigate challenges more confidently and stay motivated in your journey towards better health and well-being. Remember that you are not alone, and support is available to help you thrive with diabetes.

3. Celebrating Successes and Staying Positive

I. Recognizing Achievements:

Celebrating successes, no matter how small, is essential for maintaining motivation and momentum in your diabetes management journey. Whether you've achieved your target blood sugar levels, adhered to your medication regimen, or made positive lifestyle changes, take time to acknowledge and celebrate your accomplishments.

Keep a Diabetes Journal: Consider keeping a diabetes journal to track your progress, set goals, and record achievements. Reflecting on your successes can provide a sense of accomplishment and serve as a reminder of how far you've come in managing your diabetes.

Cultivating a Positive Mindset:

Maintaining a positive attitude is crucial for navigating the ups and downs of living with diabetes. Adopting a positive mindset can help you approach challenges with resilience, optimism, and determination.

Practice Gratitude: Cultivate gratitude by focusing on the things you're grateful for in your life, despite the challenges posed by diabetes. Gratitude can shift your perspective, increase resilience, and foster emotional well-being.

Affirmations and Visualization: Use affirmations and visualization techniques to reinforce positive beliefs about yourself and your ability to manage diabetes effectively. Visualize yourself achieving your health goals and overcoming obstacles with confidence and determination.

II. Seeking Support and Encouragement:

Surround yourself with a supportive network of friends, family, healthcare professionals, and fellow individuals living with diabetes. Lean on your support system for encouragement, motivation, and guidance during challenging times.

Join Diabetes Support Groups: Consider joining diabetes support groups, either in person or online, where you can connect with others who understand what you're going through. Sharing experiences, advice, and encouragement with peers can provide valuable support and camaraderie.

Embracing Self-Care:

Prioritize self-care practices that nourish your mind, body, and spirit. Engage in activities that bring you joy, relaxation, and fulfillment, such as hobbies, exercise, spending time in nature, or practicing mindfulness.

Set Realistic Expectations: Be gentle with yourself and set realistic expectations for your diabetes management journey. Understand that setbacks may occur, but each day presents an opportunity to learn, grow, and make progress towards your health goals.

By celebrating successes, maintaining a positive mindset, seeking support, and embracing self-care, you can navigate the challenges of managing type 2 diabetes with resilience, determination, and optimism. Remember that you are capable of overcoming obstacles and achieving your health goals, one step at a time.

Chapter 9

Planning for the Future

1. Long-Term Strategies for Diabetes Management

In this chapter, we explore long-term strategies for effectively managing type 2 diabetes and planning for a healthier future.

I. Establishing Sustainable Habits:

Focus on making sustainable lifestyle changes that support long-term diabetes management and overall health. Instead of adopting drastic measures or short-term fixes, prioritize habits that you can maintain for the long haul.

Incorporate Healthy Eating Patterns: Adopt a balanced and nutritious diet rich in whole grains, fruits, vegetables, lean proteins, and healthy fats. Choose foods that support stable blood sugar levels and provide essential nutrients for optimal health.

Prioritize Regular Physical Activity: Make physical activity a regular part of your routine by engaging in activities you enjoy, such as walking, swimming, cycling, or dancing. Aim for at least 150 minutes of moderate-intensity exercise per week, as recommended by health guidelines.

II. Continuous Monitoring and Adjustments:

Stay vigilant about monitoring your blood sugar levels, medication adherence, and overall health status. Regularly track your progress, identify patterns, and make necessary adjustments to your diabetes management plan in collaboration with your healthcare team.

Attend Regular Check-Ups: Schedule regular appointments with your healthcare provider to assess your diabetes control, review treatment goals, and address any concerns or challenges you may encounter.

Educating Yourself and Others:

Take an active role in educating yourself about diabetes management, including staying informed about the latest research, treatment options, and lifestyle recommendations. Knowledge empowers you to make informed decisions about your health and advocate for your needs.

Share Knowledge with Loved Ones: Educate your family members, friends, and caregivers about diabetes and how they can support you in managing the condition. Open communication and understanding can strengthen your support network and improve diabetes management outcomes.

III.   **Setting Realistic Goals:**

Set achievable and realistic goals for managing your diabetes and maintaining overall health. Break larger goals into smaller, manageable steps, and celebrate each milestone along the way.

Focus on Progress, Not Perfection: Embrace a growth mindset and recognize that managing diabetes is a journey with ups and downs. Celebrate progress, no matter how small, and learn from setbacks to continue moving forward.

Building Resilience and Adaptability:

Cultivate resilience and adaptability to navigate the challenges and uncertainties that may arise in managing diabetes over the long term. Develop coping strategies, seek support when needed, and maintain a positive outlook even in the face of adversity.

By implementing these long-term strategies for diabetes management, you can proactively plan for a healthier future and optimize your overall well-being. Remember that managing diabetes is a lifelong journey, and by prioritizing sustainable habits, continuous monitoring, education, goal setting, and resilience, you can take control of your health and thrive despite the challenges posed by the condition.

2. Planning for the Future

Preventing Diabetes Complications

In this chapter, we delve into the crucial aspect of preventing diabetes complications and planning for a healthier future despite the challenges posed by type 2 diabetes.

I.   **Understanding Diabetes Complications:**

Diabetes can lead to various complications that affect different organs and systems in the body. These complications may include cardiovascular disease, neuropathy, nephropathy, retinopathy, foot problems, and more.

II.   **Recognizing the Signs and Symptoms**

Be vigilant about recognizing the signs and symptoms of diabetes-related complications, such as chest pain, shortness of breath, numbness or tingling in the extremities, changes in vision, and wounds that are slow to heal.

III.   **Adopting a Comprehensive Approach to Prevention:**

Focus on Comprehensive Diabetes Management: Embrace a holistic approach to diabetes management that addresses not only blood sugar control but also other risk factors for complications, such as high blood pressure, high cholesterol, obesity, and smoking.

Managing Cardiovascular Risk Factors: Take proactive steps to manage cardiovascular risk factors by adopting heart-healthy lifestyle habits, including a balanced diet, regular physical activity, smoking cessation, stress management, and adherence to prescribed medications.

IV.   **Maintaining Optimal Blood Sugar Control:**

Strive for Optimal Blood Sugar Levels: Aim to achieve and maintain optimal blood sugar control through regular monitoring, medication adherence, healthy eating, physical activity, and stress management. Keeping blood sugar levels within target ranges can help reduce the risk of diabetes-related complications.

Individualized Treatment Plans: Work closely with your healthcare provider to develop an individualized diabetes management plan tailored to your unique needs, preferences, and health goals. Regularly review and adjust your treatment plan as needed to optimize diabetes control and prevent complications.

V.   **Monitoring and Managing Blood Pressure and Cholesterol:**

Control Hypertension: Monitor your blood pressure regularly and take steps to control hypertension through lifestyle modifications and, if necessary, medication therapy. Keeping blood pressure within target ranges can help reduce the risk of cardiovascular complications.

Manage Cholesterol Levels: Monitor your cholesterol levels and work with your healthcare provider to manage them through dietary changes, physical activity, medication therapy, and other interventions. Controlling cholesterol levels is essential for reducing the risk of heart disease and stroke in individuals with diabetes.

VI.   Preventing Foot Complications:

Practice Foot Care: Take proactive measures to prevent foot complications by inspecting your feet daily for cuts, sores, blisters, or other abnormalities. Keep your feet clean and dry, wear comfortable, well-fitting shoes, and avoid going barefoot to reduce the risk of foot injuries and infections.

Seeking Prompt Medical Attention: Promptly address any foot issues or injuries by seeking medical attention from a healthcare professional specializing in diabetic foot care. Early intervention can prevent complications and promote optimal foot health.

By prioritizing prevention and adopting a proactive approach to diabetes management, you can reduce the risk of complications, improve overall health outcomes, and plan for a future filled with vitality and well-being despite living with type 2 diabetes. Remember that prevention is key, and by taking control of your health today, you can enjoy a healthier tomorrow.

3.   Resources for Ongoing Support and Education

In this chapter, we explore the importance of accessing resources for ongoing support and education to empower individuals living with type 2 diabetes to proactively manage their condition and plan for a healthier future.

I.   Importance of Ongoing Support and Education:

Recognizing the Need for Continuous Learning: Living with type 2 diabetes requires ongoing education and support to stay informed about the latest developments in diabetes management, treatment options, lifestyle recommendations, and self-care practices.

Addressing Information Gaps: Many individuals with diabetes may encounter information gaps or misinformation about their condition. Accessing reliable resources for education and support can help fill these gaps and empower individuals to make informed decisions about their health.

II.   Utilizing Diabetes Education Programs:

Benefits of Diabetes Education Programs: Diabetes education programs offer valuable resources and support to individuals living with type 2 diabetes, including information about diabetes management, healthy lifestyle habits, medication management, blood sugar monitoring, and coping strategies.

Finding Accredited Programs: Seek out accredited diabetes education programs offered by healthcare facilities, community organizations, or online platforms. These programs are led by certified diabetes educators and provide evidence-based information and support tailored to individual needs.

III.   Engaging with Peer Support Groups:

Peer Support Benefits: Peer support groups provide a supportive environment where individuals with diabetes can connect with others facing similar challenges, share experiences, exchange tips and advice, and offer mutual encouragement and understanding.

Online and In-Person Groups: Explore both online and in-person peer support group options to find a format that best suits your preferences and comfort level. Online forums, social media groups, and community-based support groups offer opportunities for connection and support.

IV.   Accessing Reliable Online Resources:

Reliable Diabetes Websites: Utilize reputable online resources and websites dedicated to diabetes education and support, such as those provided by diabetes organizations, medical institutions, government agencies, and advocacy groups.

Evaluating Information: Exercise caution when accessing online health information and critically evaluate the credibility and reliability of sources. Look for evidence-based content written or reviewed by healthcare professionals or experts in the field.

V.   Engaging with Healthcare Providers:

Importance of Regular Check-Ins: Maintain open communication with your healthcare team and schedule regular check-ins to discuss your diabetes management plan, address concerns or questions, and receive guidance and support.

Collaborative Decision-Making: Actively participate in collaborative decision-making with your healthcare provider to tailor your diabetes management plan to your individual needs, preferences, and goals.

By leveraging resources for ongoing support and education, individuals living with type 2 diabetes can enhance their knowledge, skills, and confidence in managing their condition effectively. These resources provide valuable guidance, encouragement, and empowerment to navigate the challenges of diabetes and plan for a healthier, more fulfilling future.

Chapter 10

Conclusion

1. Recap of Key Takeaways

As we conclude our journey through "Managing Type 2 Diabetes: Practical Strategies for a Healthier Lifestyle," let's reflect on the key takeaways that can empower individuals to take control of their health and well-being.

I.   Embracing Lifestyle Changes:

Lifestyle modifications, including diet, exercise, stress management, and adequate sleep, play a pivotal role in managing type 2 diabetes and promoting overall health.

By making sustainable lifestyle changes, individuals can improve blood sugar control, reduce the risk of complications, and enhance their quality of life.

II.   Understanding Diabetes Management:

Type 2 diabetes requires a comprehensive approach to management, involving medication, dietary adjustments, physical activity, and regular monitoring of blood sugar levels.

Education and self-awareness are crucial components of effective diabetes management, empowering individuals to make informed decisions about their health and treatment options.

III.   Building a Support System:

A strong support network, including healthcare providers, family members, friends, and peer support groups, can provide invaluable encouragement, guidance, and motivation on the journey with diabetes.

Seeking out reliable resources for ongoing education and support, such as diabetes education programs, online forums, and reputable websites, can further enhance one's ability to manage diabetes effectively.

IV.   Setting Realistic Goals:

Setting achievable goals and celebrating small victories along the way can boost confidence and motivation, making it easier to sustain long-term lifestyle changes.

By focusing on progress rather than perfection, individuals can maintain a positive mindset and stay committed to their health goals.

V.   Planning for the Future:

Proactive planning for the future involves taking steps to prevent diabetes complications, accessing resources for ongoing support and education, and engaging in regular communication with healthcare providers.

By prioritizing preventive measures and staying informed about the latest developments in diabetes management, individuals can optimize their health outcomes and enjoy a fulfilling life despite diabetes.

In closing, "Managing Type 2 Diabetes: Practical Strategies for a Healthier Lifestyle" serves as a comprehensive guide to empowering individuals with the knowledge, tools, and support needed to thrive while living with type 2 diabetes. By implementing the strategies outlined in this book and embracing a proactive approach to health and wellness, individuals can take charge of their diabetes journey and lead fulfilling lives. Remember, you are not alone on this journey, and with the right resources and mindset, managing type 2 diabetes is entirely achievable.

2. Empowering Yourself for Lifelong Health

In the culmination of "Managing Type 2 Diabetes: Practical Strategies for a Healthier Lifestyle," we arrive at a pivotal moment of empowerment—one where individuals can harness the knowledge and strategies within this guide to embark on a journey towards lifelong health and well-being.

I.   Embracing Personal Empowerment:

Empowerment begins with the realization that one possesses the agency to shape their health outcomes, despite the challenges posed by type 2 diabetes.

By adopting a proactive mindset and taking ownership of their health journey, individuals can cultivate a sense of self-efficacy that drives positive change and fosters resilience in the face of adversity.

II.   Cultivating Healthier Habits:

Sustainable lifestyle changes lie at the heart of effective diabetes management and overall well-being.

Through a commitment to balanced nutrition, regular physical activity, stress management, adequate sleep, and other healthy habits, individuals can optimize their health and mitigate the impact of diabetes on their lives.

III.   Building a Supportive Network:

Surrounding oneself with a supportive network of healthcare providers, family members, friends, and peers can provide invaluable encouragement, guidance, and accountability.

Seeking out support groups, educational resources, and online communities dedicated to diabetes management can further enhance one's ability to navigate the challenges of living with diabetes.

IV.   Striving for Continuous Improvement:

Lifelong health is not about achieving perfection but rather embracing progress and growth along the way.

By setting realistic goals, tracking progress, and making adjustments as needed, individuals can continue to evolve and adapt their diabetes management strategies to suit their evolving needs and circumstances.

V.   Looking Towards the Future:

Empowerment extends beyond the present moment, encompassing a proactive approach to future health and well-being.

By prioritizing preventive measures, staying informed about advancements in diabetes management, and actively engaging in ongoing self-care, individuals can lay the groundwork for a future marked by vitality, resilience, and fulfillment.

In essence, "Managing Type 2 Diabetes: Practical Strategies for a Healthier Lifestyle" serves as a catalyst for personal transformation—a roadmap to empowerment that empowers individuals to take control of their health destiny and embrace a future filled with vitality, resilience, and joy. As you journey forward, remember that the power to shape your health and well-being lies within you, and with each step you take, you are empowering yourself for a lifetime of health and happiness.

ABOUT THE AUTHOR

About The Author Dr. Maggie Alkaline

Dr. Maggie Alkaline is a passionate advocate for holistic health and wellness, specializing in diabetes management and preventive care. With over a decade of experience in the medical field, Dr. Alkaline has dedicated her career to researching, writing and empowering individuals to take control of their health through lifestyle modifications, disease prevention, dietary changes, and personalized treatment plans.

As a board-certified endocrinologist, Dr. Alkaline combines her expertise in diabetes management with a compassionate approach to patient care. She believes in the importance of education, empowerment, and support in helping individuals navigate their health journey and achieve optimal well-being.

Dr. Alkaline is committed to staying at the forefront of medical research and advancements in diabetes care. She regularly participates in conferences, seminars, and continuing education programs to ensure that her patients receive the highest standard of care.

This certificate confirms that Dr. Maggie Alkaline has successfully earned a Doctor of Medicine (M.D.) Dr. Alkaline has undergone rigorous academic training and clinical rotations focused on the diagnosis, treatment, and management of endocrine disorders, including diabetes mellitus.